Care of the

TEETH & MOUTH

Care of the
TEETH & MOUTH

Edited by
Christopher N Burchett

PILGRIMS

PILGRIMS PUBLISHING
◆Varanasi◆

CARE OF THE TEETH AND MOUTH
Pilgrims Publishing

Published by:
PILGRIMS PUBLISHING

An imprint of:
PILGRIMS BOOK HOUSE *(Distributors in India)*
B 27/98 A-8, Nawabganj Road
Durga Kund, Varanasi-221010, India
Tel: 91-542-2314059, 2314060, 2312456
Fax: 91-542-2312788, 2311612
E-mail: pilgrims@satyam.net.in
Website: www.pilgrimsbooks.com

PILGRIMS BOOK HOUSE (New Delhi)
9 Netaji Subhash Marg, 2nd Floor
Near Neeru Hotel, Daryaganj, New Delhi 110002
Tel: 91-11-23285081
E-mail: pilgrim@del2.vsnl.net.in

Distributed in Nepal by:
PILGRIMS BOOK HOUSE
P O Box 3872, Thamel,
Kathmandu, Nepal
Tel: 977-1-4700942, Off: 977-1-4700919
Fax: 977-1-4700943
E-mail: pilgrims@wlink.com.np

Edited by Christopher N Burchett
Cover design by Sasya
Layout by Asha

ISBN: 81-7769-130-9

Printed in India at Pilgrim Press Pvt. Ltd. Lalpur Varanasi

CONTENTS

INTRODUCTION TO THE NEW EDITION

"The mouth is the gateway to the body." This statement in itself gives us an idea of the importance of the function of the oral cavity. It is through the mouth that we are able to ingest the body's necessities and so it is of vital importance that it should be as free from infection as is humanly possible. Clean teeth and pure breath are the first impression that we make when we meet anybody. Toothpaste companies usually spend millions just to impress on us how clean their products make our teeth, and how fresh they make our breath. Multimillion industries have evolved around the necessity to keep our mouths anti-septic.

This book will give you a few tips on how to keep your mouth and your teeth safe by using simple and very inexpensive methods. Obviously it becomes absolutely essential that we learn something of the working of the oral cavity before we can honestly say that we know how to look after it. This book gives us a detailed description of the construction of the teeth.

As with the birth of a child it may surprise you to know that our teeth actually begin their development in the womb. There are many opinions as to how to develop strong teeth but most seem to concur that in the initial stages of life breast-feed babies develop stronger teeth than those which are bottle fed. The choice of basic foodstuffs too plays a major role in the development of sound teeth. It is also true that the surroundings and environment in which we grow up as well as hereditary factors also play a decisive role in the development of a sound and healthy mouth.

The life styles that people adopt and their choice of food often relate to their position in life. It is all too easy to sermonise and tell others not to do this or that, but we do have to consider their financial and personal situations. It would be unfair to castigate persons for not adopting the same beliefs that we have without truly understanding their problems also. This book basically deals with the do's and don't's involved when we talk about preserving our teeth and our health in general.

By realising that the mouth is a source of infection for the whole body it becomes patently clear that the more careful we are about its cleanliness the less chances arise for succumbing to disease. This book points out that the right selection of food and proper attention paid to oral hygiene are an essential part of our everyday life. Looking after one's teeth should always be a priority, for healthy teeth pave the way for a healthy body, and progressively from a healthy body to a healthy mind.

Christopher N Burchett,
February 2003,
VARANASI.

INTRODUCTION

A few words are necessary to prove the necessity of publishing this pamphlet, which has been mainly compiled from various books and journals. A large number of the reading public of India has little knowledge of how the teeth should be preserved. Indians do not generally read books on physiology and hygiene—especially dental and oral hygienic rules. The big illustrated books on the subject are too costly and voluminous and only doctors and medical students keep or study them. The English pamphlets on the Care of the Teeth, issued from England and the U. S. A., are not cheap, and are not within easy reach of the Indian reader. Therefore, a small book on the subject is a desideratum in India.

If a few persons can derive any benefit by reading this book and by acting upon the rules laid down herein, I shall feel that my labours in its compilation have been amply compensated.

Any suggestion on this subject will be thankfully received and carefully considered.

CHAPTER I

FACTS AND SAYINGS ABOUT THE TEETH

"Every tooth in a man's head is more valuable than a diamond."—Don Quixote.

"I would rather teach the Mexican people the use of a tooth-brush than to handle a gun."—President Obrigon of Mexico.

"Clean teeth do not decay."

"Millions of working weeks are lost each year through illness due to defective teeth."

"Take care of your teeth and your teeth will take care of you."

"You need never lose a tooth."

"Prompt attention to decayed teeth saves money and suffering."

The mouth is the gateway of the body."

"Our set of teeth is like a precious garland of pearls; if you lose one tooth, the beauty and the utility of the garland will be impaired."

"Seventy per cent of diseases enter the body through the mouth and that alone is enough reason why the gateway should be looked after carefully."

"The teeth begin to form in the womb from the fortieth to the forty-fifth day of the intra-uterine life, i.e., when the embryo is in the womb."

"If the expectant mother is ill, the teeth of her child will be badly formed."

"Bottle-fed children often have bad teeth."

"A clean, healthy mouth is the best insurance against disease."

Teeth are perfectly formed only in healthy children. Good food, fresh air, sunlight and exercise are necessary to the health of the child in the widest sense and especially for the formation of sound teeth. There is proof that many serious bodily diseases are directly due to a septic mouth, and could have been avoided if proper care had been taken in time. It is no exaggeration to state that millions of people around the world both from developed and developing countries have been suffering from various diseases of the teeth on account of not cleaning them properly and of their ignorance (or in some coses sheer negligence, of the hygienic principles regarding teeth.

In Europe and America even though the knowledge of dentistry has advanced to a great extent still people are carelees of how they treat their teeth. There are many dental schools and colleges in those continents, and many books and monthly journals on dental science and hygiene are being issued. The people of India cannot get proper relief from dental diseases, until a larger number of qualified Indian dentists spread throughout the country.

Most people of India apply the medicines of quacks, or generally get their painful (but sound) teeth extracted by such doctors as have little practical knowledge of the teeth, and do not know which of the teeth should be preserved and which to be extracted. If on account of any disease or pain of the gums, sound teeth are extracted, not only are those teeth lost for ever, but the after effect on the nervous system is very bad, therefore no tooth should be extracted without the advice of a qualified dentist. Extraction of a sound tooth would injure the eyes.

"Mishi:—It is a preparation of mercuric oxide—and is highly astringent. It makes the spongy gums better, but it stains the teeth an ugly black and hence its use is to be deprecated. So far as I can see it has no therapeutic value."—Dr. R. Ahmed, D.D.S.

"The ancient Indians were supposed to possess excellent teeth and healthy mouths, because: —They and their children were breast-fed. They were absolute vegetarians; they lived principally on coarse, starchy food, vegetables and fruits. They enjoyed the open-air life and exercises gained in the cultivation of their fields. They adopted simple but effective hygienic and prophylactic measures.

Hard foods tend to preserve the teeth and keep them healthy. Some Indians have very strong teeth even to this day, and can chew fresh sugar cane or crack nuts without any danger of breaking their teeth. Some athletic Indians of the present time possess such strong teeth that they can raise one or two maunds (eighty kilograms) weight with them.

The ancient Indians used to cleanse their teeth with fresh thin sticks of special herbal trees, such as, Neem, Mango and Bakul. The use of dantaun, as these sticks are called, gives exercise to the jaws, and the astringent juice acts as a tonic to the gums and what is more important, the twig is used only once. It acts as a dentifrice toothbrush, tongue scraper and gum masseur, all in one.

A well-known proverb, common in ancient India was, “He who does not masticate well, is an enemy to his own life.”

The Indian women cleanse their teeth with the bark of the walnut tree. Under its action the teeth become very white, and the gums and the lips develop a beautiful red colour.

In the science of Ayurveda we find many applications prescribed to relieve pain in the teeth. One might desist from drawing a carious tooth, and it was recommended to administer aconite, pepper, pyrethia, ginger, or sulphur. Inflamed gums were washed with vinegar. The use of extracts of myrabolam (*harh*) for spongy gums is a very ancient prescription of ayurvedic medicine and is surprisingly efficacious, also the warm oil of unripe olives and the juice of purstain or figs. An application of hot poultices on the cheek for violent pain was resorted to, or holding in the mouth of hot liquid prepared with poppy head or hyoscyamus leaves, changing it frequently. Garlic was used much in Indian food both as a spice and for its medicinal properties—"Indian Dental Journal", July to Sep.1929.

CHAPTER II

STRUCTURE AND FUNCTIONS OF TEETH

Structure—Each tooth has a crown a neck and a root consisting of one or more fangs. The crown is the part, which protrudes beyond the gum into the mouth. The neck is that slightly constricted portion which is embraced by the gum; and the fang or fangs include all that part of the tooth, which penetrates into the jawbone.

General Form—If we examine our teeth we shall notice that they vary much in general form. Those in the front of each jaw are provided with sharp, chisel like edges, and are consequently well adapted for biting or cutting; these are called the incisors. Next to these, on each side, is a single tooth of about the same size, which has a somewhat pointed crown. This is called the canine or dogtooth, because its position in the human skull corresponds with that of the long conical, tearing tooth in the skull of the dog and other carnivorous or flesh-eating animals. The human canine tooth may also be said slightly to resemble that of a carnivorous animal in general form as much as its summit is more or less conical. Beyond these canine teeth on either side is a pair of pre-molars or bicuspids, so called because each has two cusps or ridges on the top of the crown, separated by a furrow. Beyond these again are larger teeth, each possessing two or more fangs, and having a very broad and irregular surface well adapted for the grinding of foods, hence these teeth are called the molars or grinders.

A child of about six years possesses twenty teeth, called the temporary or milk teeth. These consist of four incisors in the front of each jaw, a single canine tooth on each side of these incisors and a pair of molars on each side beyond the canines. At the age of about seven years these milk teeth begin to be cast off, their places being taken by the permanent teeth which grow beneath them; and, at about the age of twelve, all have in this way given place to the permanent set. The adult possesses thirty-two permanent teeth. They consist, of four incisors, two canines, four bicuspids or pre-molars, and six molars in each jaw. The last of the molars are called the wisdom teeth; they do not appear till between the seventeenth and twenty-fifth years.

The mass of tooth consists chiefly of a hard substance called dentine or ivory. It resembles in composition the compact tissue of bone, but contains a much larger proportion of mineral matter, and is consequently harder. The mineral matter, like that in bone, consists chiefly of calcium phosphate and calcium carbonate; and the animal matter may also be made to yield gelatine by boiling.

Inside the tooth there is a cavity, which is called the pulp cavity. It contains a very soft substance, the pulp. This consists of a mass of minute blood vessels and nerves, which enter through an opening at the point of each fang.

The dentine, which forms the crown of the tooth covered with a substance called the enamel. It is the hardest substance in the body, and contains only two or three per cent of animal matter. A substance called the cementum surrounds the root of each tooth. This substance is softer than the dentine and in structure resembles bone.

Functions—The use of the teeth is to masticate the food, that is, to reduce it to such a finely divided state that it may be readily acted on by the various digestive fluids. It has already been noticed that the different kinds of teeth are adapted for different modes of action; and we may now observe how the complex movement of the lower jaw still further increases this variety of action. When we bite our food we move the jaw perpendicularly, and make use of the front or incisor teeth. After this, it is passed over to the molars, which thoroughly crush and grind it. Now this grinding could not be carried on effectually if the lower jaw were capable of a vertical motion only. But if we observe the motion of the jaw during the grinding of the food, we shall find that it moves a little to the right and left, and also forward and backward. The broad and rough surfaces of the molar teeth are consequently caused to slide over each other, thus thoroughly grinding the food, which may be between them.

During mastication the food must be continually moved about, so that every portion of it may be brought between the molar teeth. The muscles of the tongue, cheeks and lips affect this. The action of the muscles concerned in mastication would generally be regarded as a voluntary action; but it is often partly or wholly an involuntary act, since it not infrequently continues for sometime while we give no thought whatever to it.

Mastication—The teeth are arranged precisely in the order of the work: the cutting teeth in the front—just to take into the mouth the portion desired, and separate it from the piece in hand; the tearing teeth—working the meat into a rough sort of pulp; the larger flat surface teeth at the back, the grinders—reducing still further the total mass of food. Then you would notice that it is a "wet" process, for the mouth is full of saliva; and this blends with and softens the food. But more than this, there is in the saliva a digestive enzyme for dealing with starch, and if we would only masticate more thoroughly and eat more slowly, this enzyme would save a good deal of digestive labour at a later stage. The enzyme is secreted with the saliva; and although small in quantity is potent in quality. The mouth then being the first stage—really the first opening to the stomach—deserves more care than it generally gets. Not only should the teeth be kept clean but also the mouth itself; a rinse night and morning, or better still, after every meal, with a pleasant antiseptic solution would help us all. The taste buds or nerves of the tongue have something to say about this: only with a clean mouth will they be able to give us all the pleasure the taste can afford. And taste helps digestion, for the pleasanter the taste the longer the food remains in the mouth and the more the mouth can do.

CHAPTER III

RULES OF HYGIENE

The bone of the jaw to which the teeth are attached is soft at baby age and often becomes deformed because of some bad habit, such as, the child sucking a finger or a thumb or a comforter. Children who breathe through their mouths, instead of the nose, often have deformed jaws. If children eat hard food and grind it well, their jaws will grow.

If the food is fibrous in nature, and if it is well chewed, then the regular arrangement of the teeth allows them to be cleaned naturally. Under such conditions the teeth are cleaned at every meal and hence they do not decay. Crumbs of bread, biscuit, and potato, etc., decompose and form acids, which are the cause of the first stage in the decay of the teeth. This decomposition takes place more readily at night, for the crumbs remain undisturbed when we sleep.

Modern foods are as a rule too pulpy or soft; a certain amount of hard, coarse food is essential, not only for the exercise of our jaws and teeth, but also to counteract constipation. In order to give exercise to our gums and teeth, we should properly chew sugar-cane, almonds, walnuts, cocoanuts, flattened rice or roasted rice, raw or roasted gram, mung, oats, peanuts or similar other articles. Even pressing the upper molar teeth over the lower ones or chewing beetle-nuts (paan) or datuan (i.e., green twigs) will give exercise to a certain extent.

When cleaning the mouth with water, we should force out the water through our teeth, so that the particles of food lodged in the cavities between the teeth may be forced out. Sometimes we should try to force out such particles by means of forced air or saliva with the help of our tongue. We should anyhow clean the inter-spaces between the teeth very carefully. Dirty teeth are very repulsive; not only do they look bad, but also they invariably make the breath foul and ruin health.

The food we eat should be properly chewed before swallowing. We should remember that the stomach has no teeth to grind food. By proper mastication the food has mixed with saliva, which is a great solvent. If not properly mixed with saliva the food takes more time to digest. Some animals ruminate their food by taking it out from their stomach, in order to chew it properly and mix with saliva. Masticate your food so as to mix it with saliva till you feel a sweetening taste. Do not break walnuts or almonds or whole beetle-nuts with your teeth.

The more completely the food is separated up into small portions, the more easily will the digestive fluids reach every particle of it and the more thorough and speedy will digestion be. The disadvantage then, of "bolting the food" ought to be apparent. If the breaking down process is not accomplished in the mouth it has to be performed by the stomach, and the stomach has no apparatus for such a purpose. All persons, children in particular, who are very prone to swallow their food without chewing it, should be trained to take time to do this part of the their eating thoroughly.

A massage of the gums, morning and night, will tend to stimulate the blood flow in the gums. With the forefinger and thumb gently and firmly grasp the gums well above the necks of the teeth and press towards the chewing surface of the teeth. The tongue can also easily massage the gums, especially their inside, several times a day. By such massage the pus in the gums of rotten teeth can be removed.

Chewing of tobacco leaves with lime, corrodes the teeth, reduces the sensitiveness of the tongue and discolors the teeth, gums and lips. Smoking of tobacco, cigars and cigarettes produces the above defects in a lesser degree. Therefore, these bad habits should be avoided.

Gumboils are the result of poisons from the dead nerves, or pulp of a neglected tooth. They produce pus continuously. Pus is a deadly poison. Indigestion, anemia, lowered vitality and even death frequently result from the continual swallowing of pus from these "pus factories."

The commonest cause of toothache is a decayed or decaying tooth, a gumboil at he root of a tooth. Or frequently a disordered stomach, especially among children.

Paan chewing is very bad for the teeth and gums. It helps to form tartars and causes recession of the gums, and in the course of time surely leads to pyorrhea. One, two or three pans a day may be tolerable, for the fact that paan is an antacid, deodorant and carminative. Paan stains the teeth and mouth with an ugly red, and what is worse, causes an enormous waste of saliva.

It has been proven that diseased teeth are the indirect cause of many serious illnesses—tuberculosis, diabetes and even cancer. Even, if not seriously ill, a man or a woman with a septic mouth suffers in health. Their skin looks dirty; their breath is foul; they have indigestion, they are languid and are always complaining.

Disease of the teeth is preventable if the teeth are clean, regularly inspected and decay checked early. If decayed teeth are not attended to, not only is toothache frequent, but also abscesses form and the mouth becomes the breeding ground for germs. The enamel of the teeth once destroyed can never be replaced.

Dry feeding is a system, which stands upon bedrock. Physiology supports it, instinct confirms it, reason acknowledges it, and it is anyone's to put to the proof. It is nature's way. Remember to chew, chew, chew and chew again; thorough mastication of all food is of the utmost importance to health. Take time over your meals; don't read at meals; don't eat between meals.

Preservation of the teeth also demands that the breath should be taken through the nostrils. The teeth require that the surfaces be kept in good working order. When one breathes through the mouth, the mucous membrane has a tendency to become dry, the teeth loose their needed supply of moisture and then comes discoloration, toothache, decay, looseness and finally the loss of teeth. Pressing the upper and lower jaws together very tightly in the morning just when you wake up, ensures a long life for the teeth and removes all shakiness.

MOUTH HYGIENE

Cleanliness is the foundation of mouth hygiene. Most disease germs enter the body through the mouth. Over twenty varieties of disease germs have been found in the mouth, including those of diphtheria, tuberculosis, pneumonia, influenza, and typhoid, etc.

Remove any foreign body from the hollow of the tooth, wash out the mouth several times a day with water, in which a few grains of permanganate potash, or alum, or salt might be dissolved. This removes fermentation. Permanganate of potash, and alum, etc., makes a very useful mouthwash and gargle for ordinary purposes. It cleanses the mouth and often takes away a faetid, that is, bad smelling breath.

As several diseases are infectious, and as it is difficult to know who are suffering from infectious diseases, it is not safe to use common dishes or drinking cups. The habit of putting chewed or half-eaten morsels of food or chewed betel into the mouth of children is unhygienic.

For an ordinary mouthwash nothing is better than a pure table salt and water solution. Gargles for the throat should be made with water four or five times a day, especially after each meal, in order to clear the back portion of the mouth. The object of such gargling is to clean the throat. It should be done with the neck bent backward. Forcible or loud hawking might irritate the throat—so avoid it.

The practice of kissing children and others, especially on the lips, by infected or diseased persons should be discouraged. Seemingly healthy persons might have lurking diseases. Thorough mouth cleaning in sickness—Greater care is necessary in sickness than in health, and irregular and crowded or weak teeth need much more attention to keep them in a wholesome state than those more regularly arranged and better organized.

The care of the temporary teeth—They are liable to the same causes of decay as the permanent ones, and equal care should be taken of them. It is not the design of nature that the first set of teeth shall be lost by the destruction of the crowns, but by the destruction of the roots. The parents should clean these teeth twice daily when the child is too young, and by either when the child is old enough. Children should properly wash their mouth morning and evening.

Do not turn over the pages of a book by licking your finger. It might spread contagious disease.

BRUSHING

Clean out the spaces between the teeth, first outside, then inside, then brush along the tops of the teeth, then clean the outside of the teeth and then clean the inside. After that, wash your mouth and your teeth well. The grinding surfaces should be scrubbed with a to-and-fro movement.

All the surfaces of the teeth should be cleaned outside and inside, and on the top. All the teeth should be cleaned, the upper and lower teeth of both sides, and then the upper and the lower teeth in front, and the brush should be moved from the gum upwards and downwards to get between the teeth. Brushes should not be moved too quickly, when brushing the teeth, as rough friction would injure the gums.

How to Keep Brushes Clean—The toothbrush must be kept scrupulously clean. Each person must have his own brush. Each brush must be kept separately, and in a clean place. After using a brush, it should be rubbed over soap, thoroughly cleaned with water and dried by friction over linen. Then it should be placed in the rays of the sun. Each brush must be well washed with water and soap, and preferably with an antiseptic. It is sometimes urged that toothbrushes do harm; that is because they have been allowed to get dirty and septic.

As soap is used to wash your body, so dentifrices are used to clean your teeth. As medicinal soaps are used only in special diseases, so dentifrices of medicinal nature should be avoided. All children and especially resident school boarders should be drilled in cleansing their teeth and mouth. It is important from a health standpoint to brush the teeth after each meal.

TOOTH PICKS

Toothpicks should be of the following materials and descriptions: —

Kharika (very thin stem used in Bengal), thin twigs of *neem, mango, bakul* and such other trees, quill pens, Japanese toothpicks, ivory tooth-picks, metal-tooth-picks, etc. Never use knives, needles, or pins etc., as toothpicks. Dental floss silk may also be used with advantage in some cases. If you have no crevices between the teeth and have no cavities in your teeth to catch particles of food, you need not use toothpicks.

Floss silk—The frequent passing of a thread of floss-silk between the teeth will clear away many particles that the toothbrush cannot reach. The only satisfactory way to clean between the teeth is to use dental floss silk. There are two kinds of dental floss, round and flat.

TOOTH-POWERS OR DENTIFRICES

Finely powdered precipitated chalk or charcoal, camphorated chalk, alum, ash, salt with mustard oil, camphor, etc. separately or mixed together with a few drops of carbolic acid is good. Tooth powders should be very fine and soft, and free from any gritty material that could scratch the gum. Brushing with chalk, salt or soap is useful, because they increase the cleaning power of the brush.

Camphorated Chalk Tooth Power.

Camphor —one and a half ounces.
Orris Root powder—half an ounce.
Precipitated Chalk—half a pound.
Powdered Castile Soap—60 grains
Precipitated Chalk— two ounces.
Eucalyptus Oil—sixty drops
Carbolic Acid—thirty drops
Mix thoroughly.
This tooth powder is antiseptic.

The best time to use a dentifrice is before retiring at night. During the waking hours the various movements of the tongue and muscles of the mouth in speech or otherwise, the constant salivary secretion and the mastication of food, all tend to prevent the chemical changes which during sleep take place without hinderance.

A tooth powder for a healthy mouth should be merely a mechanical agent possessing hardness sufficient for the removal of slight accumulation of food mucus, without the liability to injure the enamel; it should be slightly antiseptic and free from acidity and from rough and gritty ingredients.

Finely powdered burnt almond shells or eight parts of ordinary light wood charcoal, and one part of rock salt, is a simple, useful dentifrice. Powdered salt with a few drops of pure mustard oil will serve as a very useful dentifrice. It is easily available.

If a brush, after being dipped in water, is rubbed over a toilet soap and then the teeth be rubbed with the brush, there is no need of using tooth powder.

GARGLES

BORAX GARGLE

Borax—a quarter of an ounce.
Tincture of Myrrh—one ounce.
Water—eight ounces.

Mix the ingredients and use as a gargle for the mouth with a small quantity added to an equal quantity of lukewarm water twice daily. It is especially useful in cases of ulcers about the mouth and throat, or in relaxed sore throat and inflammation of the tonsils.

BORAX AND GLYCERINE GARGLE

Borax—one quarter of an ounce.
Glycerine—one ounce.
Rose water—one and a half ounces.
Water—four ounces.

Mix the ingredients with equal parts of water. This may be used as a gargle for sore throat, or applied full strength by a camelhair pencil, or diluted with three or four parts of water; it may be sprayed into the throat with a spray-producer for hoarseness.

MOUTH WASHES

CARBOLIC ACID AND MYRRH MOUTH WASH

Carbolic Acid—half an ounce.
Tincture of Myrrh and Borax—half an ounce.
Glycerine —one ounce.

Mix about half a teaspoonful of the mixture in quarter of a litre of warm water. It makes a most soothing and pleasant mouth wash. It is valuable for decaying teeth, and spongy gums, removes offensive odour from the breath, and is effective in removing the smell of smoke from the breath.

CHLORATE OF POTASH MOUTH WASH

Chlorate of Potash—a quarter of an ounce.
Tincture of Myrrh—half an ounce.
Glycerine—one ounce.
Water—four ounces.

Mix the ingredients and dilute with three or four parts of water. It may be used for sore throats, as a gargle, and in cases of ulcerated mouth, etc.

Limewater forms an excellent wash for weak teeth showing a tendency to decay, especially in young persons and where the saliva has an acid reaction. Limewater is alkaline and neutralizes the effects of acids.

A good mouthwash for spongy and bleeding gums is made by preparing a saturated solution of tannin in eau-de-cologne, using about half a teaspoonful to a wineglass of hot water.

DISINFECTANTS

Use clove oil, peppermint or cajeput oil, creosote, and rectified spirit. Pain in the teeth and gums can be removed by rubbing them with clove oil. Bits of myrabolam (haritaki, harh) kept in the mouth, disinfect gums.

MEDICAL INSPECTION

Unfortunately, even with the best of intentions, things can go wrong. A dentist therefore must inspect the teeth regularly every six months. The small holes can be filled painlessly and they are thereby "cured." Cavities, which are not filled, always grow larger.

When you find:—that the white hard substance called tartar has been deposited at he roots of teeth, you should go to a dentist for scraping them; that cavities have formed in them, ask dentists to fill them up; that your teeth are shaky and painful and your gums are swollen, sensitive, painful or spongy; and your teeth cannot bear a little cold or heat, go to a dentist to take out your very shaky teeth; and replace them with artificial ones; or take medicines or other suitable steps. You should take out your artificial teeth and properly clean them daily.

TONGUE

"The tongue is the natural scavenger of the mouth."

Formation of the tongue

The Tongue is a muscular organ, used for swallowing and is a special organ of speech and taste.

Size—Proportionate—The tongue with the mouth open should remain inside the teeth.

Large—Indicates suffering from indigestion.

Small—Rather rare seen mostly in the dumb.

The tongue is covered with three varieties of pimples—Thread like elevations that abound in the middle—mushroom-like elevations, scattered over the tongue. They are round and very red and the skin over them is very thin.

They contain touch corpuscles. They can at once discern the quality of what is in the mouth and whether it is too hot or cold, or just right. These pimples are longest and form a striking object at the back of the tongue.

FUNCTIONS OF THE TONGUE

The tongue and soft palate is the seat of the organ of taste. The sense of taste is excited by stimulation of the mucus membrane of the tongue and palate affecting the terminations of the nerve fibers and causing impressions to be transmitted to the brain. The substance to be tasted must be dissolved. A dry condition of the mouth is not favourable to taste and powders are not tasted till dissolved by the juices of the mouth. Acid tastes are perceived by the forepart of the tongue, bitters such as quinine by the back part and not by the fore part, sweet and salt tastes are perceived by both. It is not known how hundreds of combined tastes are perceived. Stimulation of the nerves, for example, by electricity, and without the presence of any tasty body, will excite sensations of taste. Some tastes are perceived more rapidly than others; saline tastes most rapidly of all. Flavour is a conjunction of smell and taste. One part of sulphuric acid in one thousand parts of water will be detected by the taste.

COLOUR OF THE TONGUE

The tongue is affected in most diseases. White and furred in catarrh, in affections of the stomach, and diseases accompanied with fever. To examine colour, see under the tip of the tongue by asking the man to lift his tongue.

Normal—colour is reddish.

Pale—in anaemia (poverty of blood).

Yellow—in jaundice (liver trouble).

Make sure that it is not coloured by anything that might have been previously chewed or eaten, e.g., beetel (paan), jamun, and blackberry, etc.

FUR COATING ON THE TONGUE

This coating may be white, yellow, dirty or lemon. No fur is present normally on the tongue, except in the posterior one-third portion, viz., the portion which does not touch the teeth. Whenever fur is present at the back portion it shows disease. This is very commonly seen in constipation of the bowels. In infants fur is never present.

It may be brown and dry, as in typhoid and other low fevers; often red, raw and glazed when fever is high. It is furred and flabby in dyspepsia. Small blisters are due to the bad condition of the stomach.

SECRETION FROM THE TONGUE

Normally it should be just moist, but it is unusually moist in some diseases of the mouth, salivation due to mercury poison and diseases of the pancreas. A dry tongue indicates diseases of the alimentary canal, fevers, and blood poisoning, and is found in mouth-breathers.

CRACKS, FISSURES, SCARS

Very deep fissure at the edges are indicative of syphilis, dyspepsia or indigestion. Remnants of old ulcers, etc., may be syphilitic, tuberculous or simple ulcers. Imperfect digestion and mal-assimilation are proclaimed by chapped lips coated or raw tongue, tender and swollen gums, ulcers anywhere in the mouth, bad teeth, and bad breath, etc.

The tongue is a great index to health or disease. Healthy or diseased conditions of the stomach can be detected by the examination of the tongue. Doctors generally examine the tongue.

CARE OF THE TONGUE

The tongue is a great guard of the stomach, that is, in our healthy state; the tongue by means of taste greatly indicates what sort of food should be taken and what should be rejected. Therefore, it is our duty to keep the tongue clean and healthy. Too hot or too cold, too acid, pungent, sweet or salt food or drink; strong spices or medicines and intoxicating drinks or drugs will injure the normal faculty of the tongue, and thereby pollute the saliva and consequently injure the taste discrimination, they are also very injurious to the teeth, the salivary glands, and to the stomach.

Milk and other liquid foods should always be sipped slowly, so that, it may, as far as possible, be mixed with saliva and may not cause strain on the stomach. Even water should be sipped.

A coated tongue indicates that no food at all is wanted, until the tongue is right and the breath sweet. Like other senses, that of taste may be come fatigued. Very high or low temperature deadens the sense of taste. It is the warning of nature that you should not eat or drink very hot or cold things, nor too sweet, pungent, acid, bitter, saline, catechu-like, or articles of mixed taste. When you feel uncomfortable on account of eating or drinking any article having a strong taste, gargle your mouth with water to neutralize the unbearable taste. If you take in any corrosive acids or caustic alkalies by mistake, you should drink plenty of water, milk, barley water, and arrowroot water, etc.

TONGUE CLEANERS

Tongue cleaners should be of celluloid (best cleaners), bamboo-bark (well planed), metals, etc. the upper teeth can also be used in cleaning the tongue. Tongue-cleaners should not be sharp edged.

CHAPTER IV

DISEASES OF THE TEETH, TONGUE AND MOUTH

Pyorrhea is a very common disease of the teeth. It has been estimated that about seventy to eighty percent of the people of India suffer from pyorrhea. It is generally due to lack of oral hygiene, unbalanced diet or excessive paan chewing. In all civilized countries today pyorrhea is more prevalent than has ever been known in the world's history. The cause of this is, that cooking and the artificial preparation of food were developed to high arts.

In pyorrhea gums bleed easily as a result of irritation caused by particles of food and mucus deposits when allowed to remain between the teeth. Gums are inflamed and become sore; mastication of food is difficult, constitutional health is impaired as a result of tooth and gum neglect. Mucus deposits harden and form tartar, causing the gums to recede, exposing tooth-roots. All loose teeth discharge pus from the gums, which is mixed with food and drink. The poisonous matter is constantly taken into the system, causing stomach, liver, and kidney, and bowel derangements, as well as, rheumatism and various other nervous disorders. Teeth become loose through the destruction of support around the roots. Pus pockets form; germs multiply rapidly in these pockets.

Pyorrhea is the destruction of tooth support that had taken place under sore, bleeding, receding gums. This condition results in the loss of teeth. Germs from unhealthy gums and decayed teeth cause various diseases of the body. Co-operate with the dentist in safeguarding your health. Brush your teeth night and morning. (For treatment see the end of this book)

Cracked Tongue exhibits a series of irregular furrows, of some depth, running over the surface of the tongue. They are very painful, and interfere with speaking and eating.

Treatment—Any digestive disorder, which may be the cause, should be properly treated; and borax and glycerine wash to be used freely.

Injury to the Tongue is frequently caused by accidental bites. The teeth may even be driven deeply into the tongue by a fall.

Treatment—It is best to leave the tongue alone in such a case, and to permit nature to heal the wound. Bleeding may be controlled by pressure over the part.

Cracks and Fissures of the Lips should be treated with glycerine or vaseline, the lip being kept constantly soft and moist. Cream, butter, sweet oil, oil of *til* or wax melted in the oil, may be applied over the lips.

Inflammation of the Gums—The part of gum affected is dark-red, congested and very tender. A common thing in elderly people is that condition in which the gum becomes spongy, constantly painful, and liable to bleed at the slightest touch. They separate from the teeth, which become loose in consequence. In a very large number of cases the inflamed and spongy gums are produced by the irritation of decaying stumps or small pieces of rotting teeth, or the tartar that forms on the teeth in elderly people. With their removal the inflammation disappears.

The treatment should be directed as much to the general bodily condition as to the condition of the gums. A brisk purge and hot application to the part will relieve the pain; but often nothing is equal to free lancing which permits the excess of blood to escape, and thus immediately gives relief. Sluggish action of the bowels and liver will maintain the bad state of the mouth. Free use of purgative medicines should, therefore, be made to unload the digestive organs, and astringent washes and gargles used for the mouth, those of chlorate of potash, borax, or tannic acid being the best; while a tooth-brush should be used daily with camphorated tooth-powder, the gums being will rubbed. The tongue is the best-suited organ for massaging the gums and cupping out bad blood from them.

Gumboil is usually due to the irritation of a decayed tooth. Beginning in the socket of the tooth it works its way outwards. The more deep-seated it is, and greater difficulty it has in coming to the surface, and the more intense will be the pain. Usually it is evident from the swelling of the gum, that a gumboil is being produced. Sometimes when it is deep-seated, at the end of the fang of the tooth, there is no apparent swelling. In such a case, that suppuration is going on at the end of the tooth is ascertained by firmly pressing the tooth down into its socket. This procedure will give rise to severe pain if an abscess be forming at the root of the tooth, and will thus indicate the seat of mischief.

The treatment consists in the use of hot applications, in the removal of the decayed tooth and in letting out the matter where it comes to the surface. If the tooth, that is the source of irritation, is not removed or otherwise properly treated, the gumboil is liable to recur again and again.

Toothache is due to decay of the substance of a tooth—dental caries as it is called. A long period or ill health very materially affect the resisting power of the teeth and make them easy victims to decay. Toothache is generally caused by irritation or inflammation of the nerve of the tooth. Toothache is sometimes neuralgic, i.e., affected with severe pain in the nerves, especially of the face, coming at regular intervals, and then sound teeth are attacked.

Treatment—A drop or two of weak carbolic acid or oil of cloves to be very carefully applied to the cavity of the painful tooth with pointed camelhair pencil. See that the brush does not touch the mouth, cheeks, gums or tongue. If a tooth is simply sensitive to exposure of the dentine, a mouthwash of two teaspoonfuls of bicarbonate of soda to a glass of water is recommended several times a day to allay pain. Pain in the teeth and gums can be removed by the rubbing of clove oil or keeping bits of myrabolam (haritaki, harh) in the mouth.

Stopping decayed Teeth—Scrape away the decayed and decaying parts of the tooth and fill up the cavity with some kind of cement, gold or amalgam, this is best done by a dentist.

Artificial Teeth can be fitted by a dentist to replace extracted teeth. They should be taken out after every meal and properly brushed, washed and dried with clean linen. They should be always removed at night during sleep, for they are liable to slip off and pass back into the throat.

Bleeding after Extraction of Teeth is sometimes troublesome, and even dangerous. The cavity left by the removal of the teeth should be well cleaned out. The cavity should be plugged with cotton soaked in tincture steel and pressure applied on it. A little bleeding after extraction of teeth is more or less natural.

Tartar or salivary calculus is a deposit of earthy material on the teeth at the margins of the gums. The deposit is separated from the saliva, and is mixed with remains of food. It is found in greatest abundance on the front teeth of the lower jaw and the grinding teeth of the upper jaw, because they are nearest the opening of the ducts from the salivary glands. It is an irritating substance, produces congestion and softening of the gums, which may lead to ultimate separation of the gums from the teeth and loosening of the latter in their sockets. If tartar has accumulated it should be removed by a sharp instrument if necessary, but if proper care is taken of them it will not be permitted to accumulate to a very great extent. It is best to have the teeth scraped by a dentist once every year.

Broken teeth should be extracted with the advice of a good dentist. Broken roots are often the cause of a blind abscess and should in all cases be removed; otherwise they would lead to a general lowering of health.

Extraction of a Tooth—When you find a tooth very painful or decayed or broken, or very shaky; or when a dentist says that the tooth won't work at all, then only it should be extracted by catching hold of it with fingers, or by tying it with a thread and giving it an upward or downward pull, as it is a lower or upper tooth; or it should be taken out by a dentist without giving you any pain by injecting cocaine. You should see that in no case a little defective tooth be extracted simply for temporary pain or shaking. A shaky tooth can serve you for years.

Gumboils are sometimes limited to the substance of the gums, and sometimes connected with the decay of a tooth. In the first variety it is a disease of only a few days duration, and ceases almost as soon as the boil has burst or is opened; in the second, it may continue troublesome till the tooth is extracted.

Treatment—Gumboils, when connected with an unhealthy condition of the adjacent teeth rarely disperse without passing into suppuration, and, it is, therefore, better to encourage this process by the use of warm fomentations, or poultices than to repel it. An early opening of the tumor is of importance, as, from the structure of the parts concerned, the walls of the abscess are usually tough and thick, and the confined matter seldom obtains a natural exit with sufficient freedom. A little mild opening medicine every other day will be found useful, and after the abscess has burst or been opened, washing the mouth twice or thrice a day with an astringent lotion will tend materially to make the cure permanent. Twenty grains of sulphate of zinc, dissolved in half a pint of rose water, will be a suitable lotion for this purpose.

Treatment—Take a pinch of powdered table-salt or alum, and lightly press it over the swollen gum with your finger—slimy water will come out from the part, the swelling will be reduced and the pain will be lessened. If the swelling is in the inside of the teeth, it can be reduced by constant pressure over the gum by means of the tongue and by letting out the pus by slightly puncturing the gum. Massaging the gum with fingers will also serve the same purpose. Proper movements of the tongue can extract the pus from the inflamed gum by cupping process. Pus, lying in the cavity of a gum between two teeth, can be taken out by pressing or massaging the gum with two fingers placed on the two sides of the gum.

Neuralgic pains of dental origin are due to reflected or sympathetic action. The nervous connections of the teeth themselves consist of three main branches, which ramify to almost every part of the face, mouth and head, and irritation to one branch often gives rise to pain at a portion of the nerve very remote from the source of injury. Thus the irritation caused by a decayed tooth in the lower jaw may be reflected in such a manner that the pain is experienced in the upper jaw, or vice versa.

Oral Sepsis, or Septic Mouth—Our general health depends largely on the condition of the mouth, and many diseases, including those of the most infectious or dangerous character, are due directly to a septic or unclean mouth. Septic mouth is caused primarily by neglect; even those who clean their teeth regularly. Often do it so ineffectually that the bulk of its microbic population remains undisturbed in recesses round and between the teeth, or in the folds of the common mucous membrane of the mouth.

Decayed teeth, acute and chronic abscesses— exposed pulps, dirty dental plates, badly designed crowns or bridges, inflamed gums, pyorrhea or tartar are all active factors in producing a septic mouth. Microorganisms in the mouth cause decay of the teeth, inflamed gums and pyorrhea. In the throat and lungs they produce common colds, tonsillitis, pharyngitis, pneumonia and tuberculosis, and in the stomach gastritis and gastric ulcers, and in the intestines appendicitis. They pass from the mouth through the connecting passages to the eyes, nose and ears, causing disease in these organs. They may enter the bloodstream and swarm in millions, attacking the cartilages of the joints, causing rheumatism; they poison the nerves, producing headaches, neuralgia and nervous symptoms.

Treatment—The juice of apples, oranges, and lemons will clean the mouth and throat, and remove the effects of pyorrhea.

Grinding of the Teeth by Children—Not only the act of grinding the teeth does harm to the teeth, but it is also a sign that the patient is not in perfect health. If a child is given to this habit, we may suspect, that his digestion is at fault. It may be that he has food too near bedtime, or that it is too heavy for him. Or that he has worms, a most likely cause. Or that he is of a nervous temperament, and is allowed to become too excited before going to bed.

Treatment— Attention to these matters should secure a speedy cure. When the grinding is actually proceeding, it is a good plan to turn the child on his side if he is on his back, and vice versa.

Diseases from Dental Caries—We have only recently grown to appreciate the relationship between good teeth and good health. It is practically certain that many people suffer from a number of complaints, seated far from the mouth, which are the outcome of dental caries. When we recognize that decay is a breeding ground for myriads of germs, this contention is not difficult to understand. Diseases of the blood and the nerves are the first to appear, and indigestion is bound to follow when thorough mastication is impossible.

Treatment—A person who suffers in health and who, at the same time, has bad teeth may rest assured that a thorough overhauling of the mouth will result in an improved condition of the whole body. Good health cannot continue long without sound teeth.

Inflammation of the Mouth, accompanied by the formation of ulcers on the tongue and the inside of the cheek, and decay of the gums, is specially a disease of weak children, living in ill-ventilated apartments.

Treatment—Cleanse the bowels give nourishing food. Keep them in open air. The mouth should be bathed with a solution of thirty grains of chlorate of potash to one ounce of water.

Thrush, in which small white patches are formed over the tongue, lips, throat and lining membrane of the mouth, is also a childhood disease.

Treatment should consist of giving suitable food, thorough cleanliness of all feeding bottles, and rubbing the mouth and gums with a mixture of borax and honey.

Ulcers of the Lips—occasionally form on the mucous membrane lining the inside of the lips. The ulcers are of a small circular or oval shape, of an ash gray colour, and depressed beneath the surface. They are painful, particularly when chewing is performed. They may be caused by the irritation of a bad tooth, and are frequently the accompaniment of digestive disorders.

The treatment consists in removing any cause that may exist in the form of bad teeth, and in the use of simple opening medicine, such as, Seidlitz powder, citrated magnesia, etc. the pain is rapidly relieved and the ulcer healed by applying with the finger, or camel-hair pencil, some of the tincture of myrrh and borax, or a solution of chlorate of potash (fifteen grains to an ounce of water) with a small quantity of added glycerine. A solution of the same strength of borax and glycerine or borax and honey, is also useful.

Dental Decay—Dental caries or decay of the teeth is a septic disease caused by the acid-producing microorganisms of the mouth. These germs exist in every mouth, but where the teeth are strong and the enamel well developed, the teeth are to a considerable extent immune from attack. To excite decay it is necessary for the microorganisms to remain for some considerable time in contact with the tooth substance. This is impossible between the teeth and in pits and crevices in the enamel where they are little disturbed by mastication or even by cleansing as usually performed. In such positions, which retain small particles of food, fermentation, started by the microorganisms, produces an acid, which attacks the tooth-substance, dissolving the lime salts, and leaving a thin layer of the animal matrix unprotected. They then invade the layer, and producing more acid penetrates deeper into the teeth. The germs have then established their hold and extend their activity towards center of the tooth following the dental tubuli (microscopic tubes in the dentine), which they penetrate, dissolving the lime from the surrounding dentine and enlarging the tubuli. Later the tubuli coalesce, forming cavities, which are filled with germs. This process goes on until the dental pulp, properly known as the nerve, is reached. The germs then attack the pulp which becomes inflamed and painful (toothache), and as the blood circulates through the pulp a passage is opened by which the germs may then enter into the blood stream, producing diseased conditions in parts remote from the real cause of the trouble. The bacillus tuberculosis, the germ of consumption, especially is thought to enter the system through the exposed pulps in decayed teeth. The pulp is ultimately poisoned by the overwhelming multiplication of the germs (bacteria); the tooth is then said to be "dead". It becomes very offensive owing to the putrefaction of the pulp, but it ceases to ache. After a period of quietness the microorganisms from dead pulp find their way through the foramen or orifice by which the nerve and blood supply entered the tooth and infect the socket. The tooth become tender, the swollen membrane lining the socket lifts the tooth so that it comes in contact before the others, causing intense pain in closing the jaws. The face becomes swollen and frequently the temperature rises, an abscess forms, which after a period of five to ten days discharges its pus and subsides. It may discharge externally through the face, causing disfiguring wounds, but it generally breaks inside the mouth. The tooth may then cause no pain, but a small orifice remains, generally surrounded by a slight elevation in the surface of the gum (gum-boil). From this orifice a constant discharge of pus takes place. A condition known as chronic abscess supervenes. This condition is dangerous to the general health, as the germs have invaded the living tissues beneath the tooth and they are far more likely to infect the blood than when the pulp alone is infected.

***A Warty Growth of the Lips* and its Treatment**—Its colour is white. It should be touched with glacial acetic acid once or twice daily. Care must be taken not to touch the rest of the lip. It is best applied by the end of a match moistened with the acid.

Warty Growths are also formed on the tongue.

Treatment—The acetic acid us used for similar growths on the lips, may be tried.

Inflammation of the Tongue accompanies the affliction called salivation, in which the chief feature is a continuous flow of bad-smelling saliva, which constantly dribbles from the mouth. The salivary glands are swollen and painful, and the tongue, gums and other parts of the mouth share in the inflammation and swelling. The smell from the mouth is very foul.

Treatment—Use mouth washes of chlorate of potash as previously mentioned. Use opening medicine and take three-grain doses of iodide of potassium given in water, twice or thrice daily.

Inflammation of the Tongue, with great swelling, pain, inability to speak or swallow may, however, occur alone.

Treatment—It is to be treated with brisk doses of opening medicine of ordinary salts, or Seidlitz salts. Gargles similar to those prescribed above are also to be used. Large hot applications under the chin will help to relieve the pain and the swelling.

Ulcers and acute Pain of the Tongue—Ulcers are frequent and are commonest at the sides from the friction with a decayed tooth. Smoking, too hot tea or coffee, solid or liquid foods; strong spices, acids, salts or pungent things may cause acute pain in the tongue lasting for days.

Treatment—For the ulcers of the tongue use the medicines prescribed in the 'Ulcers of the Lips'. To prevent acute pain in future, avoid the use of such articles, which cause the pain.

Bad Breath—Sometimes the person who has bad breath does not detect it, because he gets accustomed to it. But the person who sits by him feels the bad smell. Bad bleeding gums or decaying teeth emit the smell. Sockets are formed and filled with pus. Decaying food between the teeth, constipation, liver and stomach disorders, smoking of cigars or cigarettes, are generally the causes.

Treatment—After ascertaining the cause, remove it. Give brisk doses of "salts" to clear out the bowels.

Nature and Treatment of Pyorrhea—The earliest symptom is a general thickening and sponginess of the gum, which show a tendency to bleed when the teeth are cleaned. Nearly all cases of pyorrhea start with the inflammation of the gums. At this stage few patients worry their heads about the care of the mouth, because it is not painful. Discoloration, which is the forerunner of tartar, begins at the gum margin and causes irritation and inflammation, which in the earlier stage is slight and the inflammatory exudation finds its way into the mouth; but in the latter stages the deposit gets thicker and presses against in the inflamed gums and stops the exit of the exudation which burrows into the socket of the tooth and forms pus pockets. This goes from bad to worse till the tooth gets loose and local gumboils keep forming.

The pus from the tooth sockets is an intense poison, and is continually being absorbed into the circulation, partly from the gum surface, and partly from the stomach into which it is continually being carried by the food and saliva.

Treatment of Pyorrhea—The removal of the tartar is a necessary preliminary. The utmost cleanliness must be observed, the teeth being brushed frequently, especially after each meal and before going to bed, with a soft brush and the spaces between the teeth cleaned with floss silk or with toothpicks. Common salt is of benefit in mild cases of pyorrhea. It is a mouth cleanser and has a direct and valuable hardening effect on the gums. Application, once a day, with a drop of lemon juice on the brush is sufficient. Common baking soda is mildly effective as a tooth and mouth wash. A pinch of soda should be dissolved in two or three ounces of water and used from three to five times a day for two or three weeks.

The tongue may be used as a means of massage for the gums by running it vigorously many times each day over the gums. The gums should be massaged with the fingers, or, if necessary, with common salt or tannic acid powder as many times as possible. Astringent mouth-washes, such as tannin and chlorate of potash, will reduce the sponginess of the gums; while the use of carbolic acid (one drachm to one pint of water), or of peroxide of hydrogen or other disinfectants, will do much to remove the unpleasantness from the breath.

The progress of the disease can be checked by treating the gum round the necks of the teeth with iodine or other agents. Oranges and other acid fruits may be rubbed directly on the gums or the juice may be squeezed on a toothbrush and used gently as a dentifrice. To keep the teeth free from pyorrhea, and firm and well able to masticate food, it is necessary to eat less meat, starches and sugary foods, and more fruits, raw vegetables and whole-grain cereals. Constipation has to be removed by proper diet, and, if necessary, by laxatives or purgatives. In the advanced stage of pyorrhea intestinal antiseptics might be used.

TREATMENT BY THE DOCTOR

All teeth, which remain functionless and are very painful for a long time, will have to be extracted. Scaling, that is, removing the tartar from even the roots in the pockets is also essential and should be done regularly. Surrounding tissues should be treated with drugs. All cavities in the teeth should be filled up. The pocket must be removed and the gums made self-cleansing by the extraction of quite useless teeth and the removal of the flap of the gum and of the outer wall of the pocket.

HOMOEOPATHIC TREATMENT

For affections of the Gums and Teeth, Swelling and inflammation—*Belladonna, Ferrum Phos.*

Bleeding of the gums—*Ferrum Phos, Mercurius.*

Fistula of the gums—*Calcaria, Silicia, Creosote.*

Abuse of mercury—*Carbo. Vegetabilis, Hepar Sulphur.*

Toothache—*Belladonna, Nux Vomica, Mercury, Chamomilla, Sulphur, Pulsatilla.*

SYMPTOMATIC INDICATIONS

Belladonna—For painful swelling of the gums, redness of the face; pulsation in the head or cheeks; dryness of the mouth and throat; with excessive thirst; aggravation at evening time, in the open air and after lying down.

Chamomilla—Violent shooting, insufferable pains, shining swellings of the gums, violent agitation and tossing; or great weakness to the extent of fainting. Aggravation or renewal of the pains after drinking.

Mercurius—Shooting pains in the carious teeth, or in the roots of the teeth; nocturnal perspiration; great salivation; discoloration of the gums, with ready bleeding and burning. Aggravation at night by the warmth of the bed; after eating or drinking anything cold.

Nux Vomica—Jerking pains in persons who habitually indulge in coffee or spirituous liquors, or who lead a sedentary and confined life. Aggravation in the morning, during a walk in the open air or while engaged in any intellectual labour.

Calcaria Carbonica—Congestion in the head. Painful tenderness and easy bleeding of the gums. Aggravation or renewal of the toothache from a current of air, from drinking anything cold, from noises and from the slightest chill.

Sulphur—Pulsating pains, which extend to the ears and head, with swelling of the cheeks, inflammatory redness of the eyes and nose. Shooting in the ears. Aggravation in the evening and when eating and masticating.

Carbo. Vegetabilis—Abuse of mercury, especially when the gums separate and bleed. Painful tenderness, especially after eating. Aggravated by contact with hot or highly salted things.

Hepar Sulphur—After Mercury or Belladonna, especially when there is painful swelling of the cheek. Great sensitiveness. Pains aggravated at night and on clenching the teeth.

Silicia and Creosote—Shooting pains with swelling of the bones of the jaw; pains which are seated rather in the jaw than in the teeth. Disposition of the skin to ulceration. Nocturnal heat, which hinders sleep Aggravation at night.

Ferrum Phos—In the beginning of pains with congestion of blood, hot swelling and redness of the jaws and cheeks.

Creosote—If the teeth are spoiled and black.

CHROMOPATHIC MEDICINE

Ordinarily people resort to extracting their teeth as soon as they get some pain in their teeth. This is wrong. Such pain can be generally removed by keeping blue-charged water (water in a blue corked up bottle kept in the sun-light at least for two hours) in the mouth for a few minutes.

MORE TITLES ON HEALTH FROM PILGRIMS PUBLISHING